Dedicated to my Lord and Savior, Jesus Christ, who allowed me to have diabetes for a time in order to realize how to care for myself; who stayed by my side through it all; giving me strength and perseverance.

For my husband, Dave who is my constant rock! He has supported me through this most difficult journey and lifted me up when I was down.

I also want to thank my friends and family who have prayed for me and given me good advice since diagnosis; I love you all.

Disclaimer

This book in no way substitutes for connections with your Doctor and their team of diabetic experts. I am not claiming to be a doctor or an expert. You must see a doctor if you suspect diabetes or if you are already diabetic.

This book is simply my experience with diabetes, how I reversed it in three months and some of the foods that I eat. What works for me, may not work for you. Your journey will be different than mine. However, this is a great place to start.

I send my blessings, love and peace as you go through this difficult trial in life.

Never give up ~ You CAN do this!

HERE WE GO !

I was diagnosed with Type 2 Diabetes on February 28, 2015. It's not a day you can easily forget. It's now July 10, 2015. I know it doesn't sound like long enough to be writing a book about overcoming diabetes, but I had some help.

I had a yeast infection that would not go away. I saw two different doctors about this problem and self-medicated when all else failed. While talking to my sister one day, I mentioned this infection and how frustrated I was. She told me that she once had this problem too. She told me that was how she found out she had diabetes.

I didn't want to hear that. I have struggled my whole life to lose weight and avoid such issues. I had done starvation diets, where I didn't eat any food for 56 days. This was doctor supervised and I was drained of three vials of blood weekly. To be sure I was in a state of ketosis, I peed on paper sticks daily. This was a good thing to me, as this meant that my body was eating fat. This is not, however, something you should force for as long as I did. I won't get into the medical end of it as I am not a doctor. Personally, I do not recommend this diet.

When I say I didn't eat any food, I did have shakes and clear broths only. This was done in a group setting and one day a girl came in to the group and "confessed" that she had put a powdered butter substitute on her hand and licked it one day. I was so angry with her for doing that, because I didn't allow myself any "treats". That's right, my mind was totally messed up to think that was a treat. After all, I sat down to Thanksgiving dinner with all the fixings and sipped on clear broth! It gets better.

My dad came for a visit and when he saw me, 56 days into my diet, he said I looked like I was dying. He was scared for me. This is the reason I stopped after 56 days, because the doctor had approved another round for me, which I was about to start.

Dad took me to a restaurant where he told me he was ordering me a lobster and some salad, with a baked potato. My mind was so messed up, that I thought I would be fat if I ate the salad. I cried as I lifted the piece of dry lettuce to my lips, knowing there was no hope that I would ever be thin. I had lost over 60 pounds in 56 days and, when I looked into the mirror I only saw fat. I never saw the loss. This is where anorexia begins; in the mind. I was not skin and bones as you would associate with anorexia, but I definitely had the mind of an anorexic at that time in my life and it only took 56 days to find me.

Although anorexia is known outwardly, first by extreme weight loss, it is accompanied by intense fear of gaining weight and a distorted perception of body weight. This is where I was. Not emaciated, but terrified of eating that piece of lettuce!

I ate that piece of lettuce, for Dad, not for me, crying as I lifted it to my mouth with my finger tips, not even wanting to touch it. I nibbled the tiniest bites you could imagine. Then I ate the salad. When the lobster came, I simply gave in and ate it. Everything went downhill for me from there, like I knew it would. You see, I have an addictive personality and it's all or nothing with me.

I abused alcohol and drugs, then gave them up completely. I was addicted to gambling and gave it up completely. My whole life I have been addicted to food and tried to give that up completely.

Unfortunately, this is the one you cannot give up completely! The hardest addiction of all to control in my experience.

While I was on that starvation diet, I was also in the gym three hours a day, seven days a week, all the while continuing the madness at home. I don't think I stopped moving very much in that time. I was obsessed. I'm amazed I lived through it. I'm amazed I lived through any of it.

God has always been my strength. He has seen me through it all and He will see you through it all as well. You see, there is good news to my story. I survived alcoholism; I survived drug abuse; I survived a gambling addiction; and I survived Diabetes!! We all have something in our lives... So, You Have Diabetes; Now what? Let me show you how I am Roc~N~Diabetes!

Since it is my prayer to not only survive this one, but thrive in my life, I dearly want to help you beat this disease. It's not just about me, it's about millions who contract this disease in their lives and don't know what to do.

As you turn the page, you will find the first "A DAY IN THE LIFE" listing, which is just as it says, one day of my meals. Your Day In the Life will be different from mine as you go, however, this is a great place to start.

<u>Before</u> you eat a new meal, <u>test your blood</u> sugar level and mark it down. Two hours <u>after</u> the meal, <u>test again</u> and <u>record it</u>. Keep a record of the date and time of each blood test, along with the glucose level number. This will help guide you in your food choices. More on this later.

*Any food with a * before it will have a recipe to go with it following the end of that particular "Day In The Life".*

Now, remember, this is not a punishment; this is a chance for you to feel great, both inside and out and to live your life more abundantly.

Jesus said, and was quoted in John 10:10, in the Bible, as saying:

The thief comes only in order to steal and kill and destroy. I came that they may have and enjoy life, and have it in abundance.

So, here we are; crunch time. Do you want to give up your life and your health to the "thief" (devil) who only wants to kill you and steal your joy, or are you ready to follow the One (Jesus) who wants you to have a life you can enjoy, and beyond?! It's your choice. And it is here, now. Do you mind if we take a minute to pray before you start?

Jesus, help me! I can't do this alone. I'm not strong enough and I know it. Forgive my sinful life as I turn it over to you, my Savior, the One I will trust from this day on. Thank you for carrying me when I can't find the strength. Thank you for your love. Amen.

Drawing and painting relaxes me. Find what relaxes you and do it, this will help keep your blood pressure down.

Fruit	Serving	Carb
Strawberries	½ Cup	6 gms.
Cantaloupe	½ Cup	7 gms.
Blueberries	½ Cup	11 gms.
Peach	1 medium	14 gms.
Apple	1 medium	25 gms.
Pear	1 medium	26 gms.
Banana	1 medium	27 gms.
Veggies		
Spinach	1 Cup raw	1 gm.
Mushrooms	½ Cup	2 gms.
Zucchini	1 Cup raw	4 gms.
Kale	1 Cup raw	7 gms.

These are some Carb counts for some of the fruits and veggies I use in my recipes in this book.

You can go on-line to find all the carb counts in your food. Please don't assume foods are low or no carb without checking. For instance, did you know that ½ cup of cooked sweet potato has 21 gms. of carbohydrates? That's a lot for a small amount of food, which I used to consider just another veggie.

I also thought eating a lot of fruit was good for me, however, as a diabetic, 1 medium banana has 27 gms. of carbs.! I took for granted eating a whole apple at a time, and a large one at that, thinking bigger was better when it came to fruits. I medium apple has 25 gms. of carbs.

Enjoy your fruit, but have ½ a serving and enjoy each bite.

After awhile, you will think you have it all down. When you get to that point, start from the beginning and count the carbs again as well as measuring everything. What you thought was a tablespoon may turn out to be a ¼ cup. Portion matters!

A DAY IN THE LIFE

7:30am
*Kale Scramble
2 slices turkey bacon
2 slices Low Carb whole wheat or multi-grain bread (17g Carb)
*top toast with 1t unrefined coconut oil + 2t no sugar added jelly

10am
Low Carb, Low or no sugar Yogurt + ½ T raw, unsweetened coconut

12:30 noon
2 slices low-carb whole wheat or multi grain bread
1t coconut oil or butter (use very rarely)
Lettuce or spinach (lots)
3 oz. **store roasted** turkey breast
*I buy one pound of turkey and divide it into 5 equal portions right away. This is close to the pound and makes it easy to grab one portion when you need one.
1 slice American cheese (If you like something else, keep it to 1oz)
*This is your sandwich
½ Cup snap peas, carrots or celery make a nice side
*more is not better..most veggies have carbs too.

3pm
1 mandarin orange or ¼ regular sized orange
1 oz Sharp Cheddar Cheese or your choice (low fat)
½ cup snap peas

5:30pm
3-4oz chicken breast, with or without skin + rosemary, thyme
¼ of sweet potato, baked
1C green beans (no fat)

7:30-8pm
3/4C Puffins cereal (I like the peanut butter flavor), DRY
*I chose this cereal because the sugar is very low

Kale Scramble

Scramble all ingredients together in nonstick pan after spraying with coconut or extra virgin olive oil.
½ C Kale
1T wheat bran flakes
¼ C Mushrooms
2T Salsa
1t Cinnamon
¼ C Egg Whites + 1 Jumbo Egg

Note: you can choose to either add no sugar added jelly to your toast,
or add 1/3 C mixed berries.

There are different types of Kale you could use in this recipe. I always look for the deepest green I can find and that is what I will use that week.

I'm fortunate enough to have amazing farms and local growers all around me. Always look for whatever is in season and fresh.

Don't be afraid to use your imagination. I picked up some amazing veggies on a roadside stand. Many people in my area grow more than enough for their family and sell the rest in front of their homes. I'm grateful for them since I do not have a green thumb.

Usually I get vegetables and fruits from a table in front of a neighbor's home with an honor box. That's right, we actually trust each other around here. I love that! I paid $3.50 for just picked veggies. A whole bunch of them! You can't beat that. Pay attention next time you're driving and see what you can find.

The zucchini I just got there is about 18" long! You can feed a family on that. This group of vegetables really inspired me to create new recipes. I hope they do the same for you.

Please don't think I'm taking diabetes lightly when I say, "So you have diabetes." I'm not. It's just that it's another chapter in your life and it's time to do something about it.

The day I was diagnosed was a terrible day in *my* life. I had gone to my gynecologist to see what she could do to help me with this infection and to see if it was something other than what the other doctor said. I also informed her of my sister's diabetes and asked to be tested. I had been tested before and it showed that I was pre-diabetic, so I wasn't concerned. Since they had an A1C to compare from last time, this test would be true. On a side note, I'd like to say, if you test pre-diabetic that is the best time to change your life. Fixing the problem before it attacks your body any further is your best bet.

Imagine you smell gas in your house and feel there may be a leak. You probably wouldn't ignore it, but get help to find that leak and fix it. If you didn't take that step, you also know that there could have been a major accident, like an explosion or asphyxia. So, why wouldn't you call in the experts when you know there is a problem with your body? I'm just saying. I wish I had thought of that.

A couple of days after my appointment, the doctor called me with all the joy of a person calling with good news. She said, "You were right!" (Like it was a good thing).... "You've got diabetes!" I just cried. I guess she was happy about us finding the truth, but to me, my world just ended.

I hung up the phone, in shock, told my husband, and went into a state of depression for about two weeks. I immediately made an appointment with my PCP, as suggested by the gyno. I was to see him in three days. My mother wasn't surprised by the diagnosis, since it ran in the family. I eventually thanked my sister for helping me find that problem before it got any worse.

I started looking things up on-line about what to eat and started eating differently even before I saw my doctor. I was feeling so bad for myself, I couldn't stop crying.

At this point I didn't want anyone's opinion or advice on the subject of what to eat because it would confuse and discourage me, so I kept it pretty secret at first. Only a choice few knew what I was dealing with, and they were mostly notified so they could pray for me. Not saying anything at first was a great choice because it allowed me to focus on me and my needs and not be scattered in my thoughts. I am the type of person who can get overwhelmed pretty easily, so I need to keep it simple and focused. You decide what will help you best.

I went to my doctor's appointment and had to actually say out loud, "I've been diagnosed with diabetes." This, of course set off the tears. It's so definite when you say it out loud. I felt defeated after all the years of dieting and exercising and failure, failure, failure.

He was kind, as he always is, and I trust him with my life. Make sure you have a doctor you trust. I was a bit disappointed that none of the doctors suggested I be tested for diabetes, but I had to let that go. Doctors have to diagnose by a process of elimination and I guess I just came up with the diabetes issue first because of my sister's advice. So, I fault no one in that.

He brought in a girl to show me how to test my blood at home. This was really happening. I was on the craziest ride at the carnival, spinning out of control and I couldn't get off! You know the one where you stand with others in a circular room, against a wall as it spins you to the point of pinning you to the wall as the floor drops out from beneath you. Yeah, that's what it felt like!

So, the girl with the blood tester, who couldn't have been sweeter or more understanding, carefully took out the fancy glucose meter, some strips and .... Bu bu bu baaa..... needles!! God knows how much I hate needles! She was sweet and kind and caring as I watched and listened. She came over and tested my blood as I cried, so terrified of the pain and what the meter would read. Do I really have to do this? Can I be done now? Can someone order a pizza?!

She took my blood test and it read 192, which was too high considering I hadn't eaten in awhile. My A1C was 9! It should be between 4.5 and 5.7 for non-diabetics. A1C is a number that calculates the blood sugar levels in your body for a total of three months. The test three months ago showed 6.1, pre-diabetic and I thought I was okay, because I ate well and exercised. Obviously, I was not eating right for my body, but I didn't know that yet. I was in a gym, being trained and coached by a dietician as well. I ate only what she told me to eat and exercised like I was training for the Olympics! I lost inches in that time, but the scale never went down. I was frustrated. In her defense, she did not know I was diabetic and neither did I.

Not every diet works for every person. It's up to us to see what works for us. It's very personal.

At this point, I am keeping my glucose levels between 83 and 107 before meals and 100 to 132 after a meal. I want to be careful not to go too low (under 70) or too high (over 180). Refer to your doctor and team of experts for the levels they recommend for you. It's a work in progress, but I'm doing great!

The girl in charge of teaching me to take my own blood tests, finished testing me, then handed me the device and said, "your turn". My turn? What do you mean, my turn? I didn't even like *her* testing my blood. I knew with everything I was that **I could not do what she was suggesting**!

I turned on the device, loaded a lancet (needle) into the torture chamber and placed the cap on it. I set it down and took out a test strip, placing it awkwardly into the monitor. Now came the moment I was dreading; I was feeling so sorry for myself that I couldn't stop crying. I could barely see through my tears as I leaned the lancing device (yes, lancing like swords), against the side of my finger and pressed the button, reluctantly.

It wasn't so bad! It didn't hurt much at all! Who knew? I squeezed my finger tip a bit, put the blood on a test strip and waited for the reading. It wasn't good, it read 210, without food in my body, which is ridiculously high, but I had the first test under my belt. This number was probably higher than hers due to my rising blood pressure dealing with this stressful situation. I was on my own now. I had to do this about five or six times a day for awhile, at home, by myself. I didn't think I could do it. I felt so alone. My next appointment would be with the Certified Diabetes Educating Nurse (CDEN).

I met with the CDEN a few weeks later and I had already started eating differently, according to diabetic standards. She taught me the science of diabetes, which for me was the turning point that set my mind on recovery. Knowing how my body works has really helped me to stay the course.

A DAY IN THE LIFE

7:30am

*French Toast with Berries
2 Slices Turkey Bacon

10am

Oikos Triple Zero Yogurt + 1/2T raw, unsweetened coconut

12:30 noon

 *Grilled Cheese & Tomato

3pm

*Peaches N Almonds

5:30pm

*Bison Tacos !!

7:30-8pm

3/4C Puffins Cereal (dry)^^

^^ You can choose any healthy cereal you like. I like this one because of its low sugar/carb content and it's variety of flavors. Peanut butter is my favorite. Keep the carbs and sugar as low as possible. You're not fooling anyone if you choose to eat sugary items, you are only shortening your life. Try to remember that and it may help you make better choices for yourself. Love yourself as much as you love those you surround yourself with.

French Toast with Berries
(This is one of my favorites!)

In a pie pan or deep dish mix 1 jumbo egg with 1/4C egg whites, 1t cinnamon, 1T wheat bran, 1-2T light vanilla soy milk. Mix well.

After your bacon is cooked and out of the pan, spray coconut oil, dip two slices of low-carb (17-18g/2slices) bread on both sides into mixture and place in pan. I then spray the top of the bread with coconut oil, for the flip. There will be extra egg mixture; just pour it over the bread. Cook on both sides until egg is cooked. (check center of bread for doneness). I splurge here with a sliver of butter on each slice.

Pour 1/4C sugar free maple syrup and ¼-1/3 C mixed berries into cup and place on side to pour over bread and enjoy!

Grilled Cheese & Tomato
2 Slices American Cheese (or 2 oz. your favorite melty cheese)
½ Sliced small tomato
Put these in between 2 slices low-carb bread and place in non-stick pan, sprayed with extra virgin olive oil. Cook on both sides until browned and remove from pan.
Open sandwich and add lots of your greenest lettuce or fresh spinach.

Higher carb option: Serve other ½ of tomato and ¼ of an orange with some slices of cucumber on the side.

I love when the cheese spills into the pan and forms a crust. This part is so delicious. You can see it on the side of my sandwich in this picture. It's crispy and full of amazing flavor. Since I don't use salt, these extra flavor boosters are most welcome.

Pears & Cheese with Crackers

Slice 1 pear in ½. Put ½ in the refrigerator for another time. Slice the remainder into thin slices so it feels like chips when you eat it. We need to fool our senses until this becomes something we love as much as we used to love our chips. (I now love this more than chips!)

Slice one, one ounce piece of cheese (I use extra sharp cheddar because it's loaded with flavor) and put it on the plate with the pear.

--->

I found an amazing cracker that I like to have with this meal. (It's not a snack, it's a meal. They all are. Saying snack could make your mind think about what you used to consider snacking. We eat 6 meals a day and each one is important.)

Triscuit is making a cracker made with brown rice and wheat. It has sweet potato and roasted onion. It is so incredibly full of flavor that I really look forward to this meal. They have other brown rice cracker flavors to choose from as well. Choose your favorite. And, as always, keep the carbs low and the sugar even lower. Have 3 triscuits with this meal.

That may not sound like much, but remember, we don't eat like we used to. We are not opening a box of crackers and eating it all without even tasting. We are nibbling and savoring and tasting every morsel so that we appreciate what we are having more and are, therefore, satisfied with less.

I used to be more focused on the food at a gathering than the people, now I'm more focused on the company, and actually enjoy my food more as I savor and mingle. Take time to stop and smell the flowers, or in this case, the food. I took pictures of the gardens at my sister's wedding when I normally would have been inhaling meatballs and pasta.

Bison Tacos

4oz Bison
(you can use ground turkey or extra lean beef instead, but please try bison at least once. It is extremely lean and I have come to love it.)

2T Salsa
Bunch of lettuce (the greener the better)
1oz cheese
3 Corn taco shells (no flour shells please)
1/2t taco seasoning

Cook up the meat and seasoning, bake the shells briefly and fill them evenly with the meat and other toppings. This is one of my favorite nighttime meals. Enjoy!

The CDEN showed me 2 vials. One was filled with a substance representing my blood on Diabetes, while the other vial represented blood without diabetes. This is your blood on Diabetes, This is your blood not on Diabetes. Sound familiar?

Anyway, the vial pertaining to Diabetic blood was explained as sluggish and coated in sugar, which caused it to flow slower. This causes us to feel tired and makes our body work so hard that eventually our pancreas will get over tired and give up. After that, the liver takes over producing insulin and so on. This disease attacks the heart as well and, I've been told, will kill you slowly if not taken care of.

I don't know about you, but if I have a choice, I don't want a slow death! That's all I needed to know in order to get serious about my health. There are a lot of pancreatic issues in my family to begin with, so this was a no brainer for me.

I started eating six meals a day. That's right, six. What a concept, eating more often. How is that going to help me?

Think of your body as a locomotive. There's a man whose sole job is to shovel coal into the furnace to keep the train moving. If he misses just one scoop of coal at the right time, the engine slows and eventually stops.

Our bodies work much the same way. Every two to three hours I need to fuel my system or I will visibly slow down; this is a sign my sugar (glucose) levels are dropping.

It happened to me one day in a restaurant. I hadn't eaten in five hours and I was feeling tired, but not realizing why. Our waitress, Melissa brought me some juice, which I had not asked for and I said, "I can't drink that, I'm diabetic, remember?" That's when she told me that the manager, Dave had noticed when he walked past our table, that I looked "droopy" and he knew my sugar was dropping. I didn't realize I was literally slouching over the table.

A couple of sips on that juice and it was like someone flipped the on switch. I perked right back up. Much thanks to the staff for watching over me.

You see, we are regulars at this particular restaurant and when I was diagnosed with diabetes, I alerted the staff of my new diabetic needs.

It's important to educate those around you of signs to watch for and what to do if they see a problem. This staff has been wonderful and cooks my food according to my needs, going as far as cooking me foods that are not offered on the menu. I'm forever grateful for them all. Thank you, also, Donny, Jess, and the rest for going above and beyond; you are all more like family to us than servers and managers.

I'm about to show you my everyday rules, but let me preface that by saying, that since I've gotten my diabetes under control, I have allowed small amounts of white potatoes back into my life very sparingly; in fact, almost never. At first I didn't have them at all.

Here are my everyday rules:

*No added salt
*No white sugar
*No white rice
*No white pasta
*No white bread
*Extremely limited amounts of white potatoes
*Move after every meal
*Get some exercise during the day
*Test blood at least twice a day
*Pray
*Never give up!!!

Now, don't get discouraged; it sounds pretty strict, and it is, but with time, it will become part of you and not as bad as you think.
Sure, I did a lot of crying at first, feeling so bad for myself that I didn't know what I'd do. These are *my* rules, and for now, yours; they may change for you.

I remember when a waitress walked past me with a cheeseburger and french fries and I actually cried. You are definitely allowed to mourn the loss of your food. You've known it a long time and had a love-hate relationship with it. It's not easy to give up such a stronghold, but it *is* possible. And, I'll tell you, without Jesus, I would not have had the strength to do it.

On that note, I'll tell you that in the beginning, I didn't have any white potatoes either. I didn't allow that in until I reversed my diabetes. Now I very rarely have a bite or two of white potato. It's my treat. Some people want ice cream, I want potatoes. I have, however, found some wonderful sugar-free ice cream products on the market. I'm very thankful for them.

Let's take one bullet at a time, shall we?

Bullet #1 *No *Salt*
I chose to cut out salt right away because I had high blood pressure. I had actually had it for quite some time, but when I was diagnosed with diabetes and learned that salt can contribute to high blood pressure , I decided to try and give it up to see what would happen. Turns out, it was a great choice for me because my blood pressure is now perfect.

If you have diabetes, you have a higher risk of health issues with the heart, nervous system and kidneys. High blood pressure is very common in diabetics which is why our risk is higher. Giving up the salt, reduced my blood pressure and therefore reduces my risk for heart disease and other issues mentioned above.

Bullet #2 *No *White Sugar*
Sugar is possibly the worst thing for a diabetic to take in. I'm not saying you can never have sugar again, but for now, please try to not eat sugar. That being said, there are different kinds of sugar.

For instance, fruit has sugar, but it's not white sugar, its natural sugar. Even so, it will react much like any sugar in a diabetic body, therefore, fruit must be limited to the proper serving size. You can refer to carb counters on-line to see the lists of how much of what to safely eat.

Bullet #3 *No *White Rice*
This is more difficult for your body to break down properly than perhaps a brown rice or whole grain such as quinoa or barley. These would be better choices for you.

Bullet #4 *No *White Pasta*
There are so many carbs in pasta! I don't even bother eating it anymore. If I did decide to have pasta, I would choose a brown rice or quinoa pasta. I do prefer to just use spaghetti squash in place of pasta if I really need. It.

Bullet #5 *No *White Bread*
This is just wallpaper paste. There's not a lot of nutritional value in white bread. Try to think of food choices as what

will benefit your body, rather than just what looks good to you.

Whole grains, wheat, rye; anything with unbleached flour is way better than white bread for your body. Still, watch the carb counts.

Bullet #6 *Move* after every meal
It is important for us to move after we eat to help metabolize our food and not allow it to just sit and turn to fat. I'm not saying go to the gym after every meal, just move.

When I go to the movie theatre I allow myself a serving of popcorn (without the fake butter or salt). As soon as I finish my portion, I move my legs while sitting in my seat for about 10 minutes. I don't move them so much that I'm disturbing people near me, just enough to not be sitting still.

Bullet #7 *Get some *Exercise* during the day
I say some exercise. The amount will depend on you. One day you can do some floor exercises at home and another go to the gym. Or you can take a bike ride or a walk by yourself or with a friend. It doesn't have to be drastic.

Your choices are for life, so if you go too gung ho on exercise right away, you may give up completely. You will feel what is right for you. Start with 10 minutes a day, then go to 15 and so on, until it works for your body. You can do this gradually. For instance 10 minutes a day for the first week.

Never give up! If you find bike riding is too hard for you or you don't like it, walk. If you don't enjoy your walks, go bowling. Find something that suits you. This is not a punishment. This is your time! Do what you find to be stress reducing and fun. Stress is really bad for diabetics, so take time for yourself, to wind down.

Bullet #8 *Test Blood* at least twice a day

In the beginning I tested about 4-6 times a day. I really needed to figure out what my body responded to. I found if I sat still too long my levels spiked and if I got too excited they spiked. Food and exercise are the two key things to monitor in order to get your numbers right.

Bullet #9 *Pray*

I give all the glory to God for my recovery. Yes, I worked hard and yes I had a lot of figuring out to do and yes, I had a great team around me, but I could not have found the strength to begin or carry on without Jesus walking along side me. Ask everyone you know to pray for strength and guidance for you. Prayer is powerful and I know that I can do anything as long as I have Jesus leading the way.

Bullet #10 *Never Give Up !!*

It would be so easy to ignore the fact that you have diabetes and continue on the path of destruction. Truly, it would be way easier than fixing the problem. However, as time goes on your body will start to have more problems and you will have to deal with them.

Any way you slice it, you cannot escape diabetes! It is there, lurking, waiting for you to make a choice. Life or death. Sounds dramatic, I know, but that's what it comes down to. You have diabetes today, next thing you know your pancreas gets tired of producing insulin and your liver takes over, it gets tired, your heart gets stressed and it's all downhill from there.

Please do something about it now. Just because there's an option of insulin for some, does not mean that makes it all better. You can't say, "I'm going to eat anything I want because I can just take a shot". It doesn't work that way. Please, choose a quality life. Now's the time. Today. Don't wait. Love yourself enough to take care of yourself.

Yellow Beet Chips

Rinse and dry beets. Slice thin, toss in olive oil, garlic powder, rosemary and Mrs. Dash, original. Bake at 350◦F, flipping over once, until they look crispy. Leave out in the air for a few minutes and they will crisp up. Enjoy!

*Use any type of beet you like. Yellow are much less messy to work with and I like them best.

TUNA SALAD SANDWICH

2 slices low-carb multi-grain or whole wheat bread (17gms/2 slices)

MIX: 1 Can solid white tuna in water (6 oz) (5 oz with water drained)
Olive oil mayonnaise 2 – 3 measured teaspoons
Sprinkle of Mrs. Dash
Celery or snap peas in the tuna
Put Lettuce on the bread with tuna mixture . Toast the bread if desired.

Cucumbers, one large strawberry (on the side)
Drizzle (and I mean barely) your favorite salad dressing.

MID-MORNING SNACK

Half a Bosc Pear, sliced thin

1 ounce Sharp Cheddar Cheese

3 Truiscuit Sweet Potato and Onion, Low sodium crackers

1 SQUASH 3 WAYS

I took one Acorn Squash and sliced it in half. I scooped out the seeds with a spoon then separated the seeds from the pulp. (Discard pulp)

I sliced half of the squash into thin pieces and left the other half whole.

Melt ¼ Cup Unrefined Virgin Coconut Oil and pour it evenly over all of the squash components. Then sprinkle cinnamon, liberally over all. Mix the slices to distribute the oil and seasoning, then separately, mix the seeds the same way.

With your hand, rub the oil and cinnamon into and around the ½ squash. Spread these out across a cookie sheet with the ½ squash cut side down.   Bake at 350 degrees F. for 20 minutes then remove the seeds from the oven.

Bake the remaining squash for 20 more minutes. Now drizzle, *lightly* sugar-free maple syrup over the slices and ½ squash. Return to oven for 10 more minutes then remove. Squash is ready!

The entire squash except the pulp and the stem which you discarded, is completely edible. The skin adds a nice chew and some vitamins.

Zucchini Chips

Slice paper thin. If your zucchini has a lot of seeds, you can remove them, but you don't have to. Drizzle lightly with extra virgin olive oil and sprinkle with rosemary, Mrs. Dash original, garlic powder and onion powder. Spread evenly over cookie sheet and bake at 350 degrees in 10 minute intervals, turning them over each time until golden brown. Let sit in air for 10 minutes to crisp. Enjoy.

*If you have extra, bake into a quiche or stir into eggs in the morning.

Italian Style Zucchini Boats

Remove seeds, by scooping with spoon from a large zucchini. (You can dry the seeds in the windowsill and plant them to grow your own zucchini) Cut into large chunks. (mine were 5" long) If you only have access to small zucchinis just slice lengthwise before hollowing out. You need 5 good sized chunks of zucchini.

Massage extra virgin olive oil into the zucchini, covering all sides. Sprinkle Mrs. Dash and garlic powder on all sides. Microwave all pieces for 5 minutes to soften. Bake shells in oven for 15 minutes at 350 degrees.

---->

While they pre-bake, mix the following ingredients together.

4 meatballs (I get mine from a pizza shop who uses crushed tomatoes in their sauce instead of a sugary, salty sauce – you can buy marinara).

2 spicy sausages (if you prefer sweet, go for it)

5 Tablespoons sauce

5 Tablespoons Mozzarella cheese

Sprinkle each of: garlic powder, onion powder & Mrs. Dash

¼ cup sliced mushrooms

Take zucchini out of oven and fill each shell with 5 equal portions. (1 stuffed zucchini is your portion)

The carb count is so minimal that I eat 1 slice of low carb bread with a small amount of butter on it with this dish.

Return the pan to the oven and cook until zucchini is fork tender. Check it every 10 minutes. Do not overcook; we're not making mush here. If you didn't like zucchini before and you cook this properly, you will love it! I never liked it before either. Top with zucchini chips if you like.

GO TO SNACK

This is one of my favorite go to snacks. ½ peach sliced super thin and one package of cinnamon or cocoa dusted almonds. They are perfectly portioned. This snack provides carbs, protein and fat and since it takes awhile to eat, I feel like I'm getting more.

Variations, of course, would be different fruits. I find ½ a pear with the cocoa almonds is a great combo.; and ½ apple with cinnamon almonds is also great.

Wherever I go, I make sure I have a food bag with me just in case there are not foods that I choose to eat at those locations. Never be caught without a backup plan. At the very least, keep a granola bar and a package of nuts in your purse, if you carry one, or in your car. This could carry you for two meals if needed.

Leftovers Crustless Quiche

Every Sunday my husband and I go out to lunch. I have educated the staff on my diatetic needs and they have been wonderful. I ask for everything on the side, not to cook my food with fat, and have asked for many things that are not on the menu and have been catered to beyond my belief. I actually call ahead sometimes and ask them to bake me some sweet potato fries.

This quiche makes my life so much easier. One quiche makes 5 breakfasts for me or 5 lunches. For breakfast I add 2 slices of low-carb (17 gms.) toast with 1tsp. coconut oil and 1 ½ tsp. no sugar added jelly. Adding a salad instead of the bread with some fruit in it transforms this breakfast into a lunch. Or simply have some sliced fruit on the side.

Here's the recipe. Spray the pie pan with Coconut or Extra Virgin Olive oil spray. Mix 5 eggs with ½ cup egg whites and ¼ cup milk. (For the milk, I use soy, but you can use a non-fat milk if you prefer) Add ½ teaspoon Mrs. Dash and ½ teaspoon cinnamon.

*Cinnamon is not sweet until you add sugar to it. It is a great spice for savory dishes as well and is a metabolism booster. It's always in my egg dishes.

Add to mixture, 1 large tablespoon of raw bran (If you have fiber issues, you can omit this). The recipe from here is all up to your refrigerator. Whatever you have in there can go in here, as long as you use proper portions. Choose 3-4oz meat, 1 tablespoon cheese, ½ cup green vegetables.

Here's what I did:

I had cooked peppers and onions leftover and pressed them into the pan to act as a crust. My mixture was poured on top of that. I used leftover steak that was topped with cheese and asparagus. For some extra carbs, I sprinkled the top with ¼ cup hash browns. These will add a crunch to the top. I don't usually use white potatoes but this is a very rare occasion. I would not use them every time, but they were leftovers in my fridge.

Bake the quiche until golden brown on top and cooked through by piercing with a sharp knife. (About 30-40 minutes) There is no crust, so it doesn't take as long. This makes 5 perfect servings. Enjoy!

HOME & RESTAURANT MEET

You will always have leftovers from restaurants if you are eating the proper portions for you. Here is just one idea.

When someone orders pizza and I know I'm going to want something with sauce when I smell it, I order 4 meatballs and 2 sausages with sauce, whole. It's important to not let them cut it up because you can see the portions better this way. That order will last me for two to three meals.

So, I put one meatball and one sausage or two meatballs and ½ a sausage on my plate. Then I make a simple salad with a small amount of parmesan cheese and 1-2 teaspoons of dressing. Then I have one or two slices of low-carb bread with ½ teaspoon of butter on each of them. Love this!

OMELETS

I love breakfast!   I could eat it three times a day, easily, but I don't. I usually have 2 slices of low-carb toast (17-18gms.) with 1tsp. coconut oil and 2 tsp. no sugar added jelly. (These are totals for both slices combined, not per slice).

I also have 2 slices of turkey bacon. I found a maple turkey bacon that I absolutely crave. Use what you like.

For the omelet you have many options. Since you already have bacon and eggs, you don't want to add any more meat. Use any veggies you like, in moderation and if you must, add 1oz. cheese.

----$\rightarrow$

One omelet combo I like includes mushrooms, kale, salsa and American cheese. Always use 1 jumbo egg and ¼ cup egg whites or egg substitute. (As long as it is made with real eggs) Scramble the eggs together and pour over cooked veggies in non-stick pan. Sprinkle cheese evenly around then fold over when cooked. Enjoy this once a day if you like. The brown spots you see in this omelet are simply wheat bran. I add a tablespoon to all of my egg dishes. Since I don't get a lot of sugar or fat in my diet, high fiber is necessary. 'Nuff said. ☺

LOVE YOUR VEGGIES

Here we have a simple coleslaw mix from a bag mixed with toasted quinoa and served cold.
The dressing is to be used sparingly.

1/2C Olive Oil Mayonnaise
1 T Extra Virgin Olive Oil
1t your favorite vinegar (I use balsamic)
¼ t Mrs. Dash, Original
*Just mix it up and use on any salad.
For the coleslaw I used a whole bag of mix with 1/4C of the dressing.

For the quinoa, use your favorite flavor. I used sun dried tomato. Prepare it according to the box instructions, then toast it in a pan for a few minutes until it's crunchy, but not too long, because it gets bitter. Sprinkle this on top of your coleslaw before serving. Only about 1 T per serving, please.

English Muffins

Watch the carb count and always check the flour in the ingredients to be sure it is not bleached flour.

English muffins come in so many flour bases and ingredients. Be especially aware of those with fruit, such as raisins. These will be higher in carbs and you will probably want to only have ½ at a time.

½ a toasted English muffin with 2T of crunchy peanut butter and 1t of no sugar added jelly with a cup of tea or coffee is a very satisfying meal mid-day or evening.

How to determine when to eat:

I tested my blood before I ate, then an hour after, then ½ hour increments. I did this after several different types of meals to get an average eating time. What you are looking for is the time your glucose is the highest after a meal and the time it comes back to a normal level.

For example:
Before my meal my glucose level was at 107 on several occasions, so at the time, that was my "normal" level. I found that at 2 hours after my meals I averaged 133. One half hour later, bringing us to 2 ½ hours after the start of my first bite, my level goes back to 107. This told me that my glucose peaks at 2 hours (perfect time to test a meal) and it was a good time for me to eat 2.5 hours after I started eating my last meal.

I tried to go 3 hours and found I was around 99, so I was still in a safe level, in fact, even better. You don't want to go too low before you eat again either. So, I've chosen 2.5 to 3 hours for my times to eat. I take in 6 small, balanced meals every day, every 2.5 to 3 hours.

The more you keep to the same times and same types of meals, the better your body will respond. Now you give it a try. It's best to try this when you have a whole day at home. Some of my meals don't raise my glucose by much, if any. For instance, 1oz. cheese and 1/4C nuts. These are great small meals.

Once you do the work, it becomes second nature. Now relax and begin.

Quinoa Coated Chicken Breasts

Remember that quinoa you cooked? Here's another use for it, so it's a good idea to make extra.

Use 3-4 oz. pieces of chicken breasts (I cut large ones in ½). Roll in whole wheat flour, then egg white, then cooked quinoa.

Place on cookie sheet and spray both sides with coconut oil. If you can't get coconut oil in a spray, use extra virgin olive oil spray.

Bake at 350∘ F for between 20 and 45 minutes, depending on the thickness of your chicken pieces and the way your oven cooks. When it is golden brown it should be done. I flip it over ½ way through the cooking time. Always check the center of one piece by cutting it to be sure there is no pink before eating it.

I paired this up with some of the quinoa coleslaw. Enjoy!

GREAT SIDES

To make this dish, which I would serve fresh, not leftover, you only need a few ingredients.

Mushrooms, Shredded Parmesan Cheese, Kale, Spinach, Mrs. Dash Original Blend & Thyme.

Saute sliced mushrooms with thyme. When they are almost cooked, push them to the side of the pan and sprinkle your parmesan cheese evenly over the rest of the pan. Watch it closely and as it starts to bubble, put the kale, spinach and Mrs. Dash on top of the mushrooms.

Within seconds, you can flip all the ingredients on top of the cheese and start scrambling them together. The reason you toasted the cheese is because it gives a nice crunch and amazing flavor to the dish. Only cook long enough to just wilt the greens.
*If you kale doesn't wilt fast enough, just sprinkle a little water into the hot pan.

Notice I didn't give you measurements. Keep the portion to about a cup, cooked. That being said, keep your cheese (which is the fat content here) to 1T per serving.

Have fun trying new things, but remember to test before and after new meals to see what works in your body.

A certain meal may work for me, but not you and vice versa. Keep trying and you will find your perfect combination. If an adjustment is needed, try removing or adding items and re-test next time you eat it. You will find your way.

MAKE IT LAST

In one picture, I showed you these very same bison tacos, assembled. Did they tempt you? Maybe you are an interactive eater, like me. I love to put my food together as I eat it. It makes it last longer and allows me time to digest in between bites.

Here I've put the meat, cheese and sauce (which is just a bit of water added to the pan at the end) in the shells and placed the veggies on the side in fancy bowls. The salsa is also portioned out into a bowl with a spoon. Keep in mind that the salsa and tomatoes add carbs, so be sure to account for that.

Now you can take one taco, put in 1/3 of the salsa, add a couple of tomatoes and stuff it to the gills with lettuce!
If you do it this way, when you're done with that taco, what do you know? There's another one! And when you're done the work of preparing and eating that one, there's another one! Your meal lasts longer and is more satisfying.

PRESENTATION

If you find yourself getting bored with the same foods and don't really have time to try new ones yet, change the way they look!

Arrange it differently on the plate; use fun plates. If your omelet is boring folded over, scramble it or fold it in quarters. You can also put it into a low car wrap and skip the toast. (When I do this I put it back in the pan to toast it) Amazing!!

Make your food look inviting, fancy and like someone really took the time to spoil you. You did! And you deserve it!

BISON BURGER

Obviously you know how to make a burger. My suggestion is that you use lean cuts of meat. I use bison. You can also choose turkey, chicken or beef. When using these meats please use 85-95% meat. 70-80% will simply have too much fat. Bison is naturally lean.
The rules for *your* burger are as follows:
3-4oz. meat
1oz. cheese (optional)
If you use ketchup, find the low sodium choice. Mustard is a great choice.
2 slices of low-carb bread/toast or 1 slice, cut in half of another multi-grain,
   whole wheat or rye.
Lots of lettuce
A couple of slices of tomato if you wish (this has carbs and is considered a fruit)   *Pickles should be used sparingly if at all and this includes relish because they have a lot of salt.*

WHO WANTS POPCORN?

3 cups Air popped popcorn
1t cinnamon
Spray coconut oil

Pop the popcorn
Spray with coconut oil (don't overdo it~ this is for flavor and stickability)
Sprinkle the cinnamon and mix it up.

If you like kettle corn like I do, sprinkle a 1/2t of truvia or your favorite sugar substitute over the popcorn.

This is a nice night time meal for watching your favorite movie.

You can have all of the three cups in a sitting if you like.

HOMEMADE CHICKEN SOUP

1 Whole Chicken (store roasted or raw)
½ bag shredded carrots
6 stalks celery (4 chopped, 2 whole)
2 large bouillon cubes (please don't use those hard squares)
1 small 8oz. can chicken stock (if you used pre-roasted chicken only)
3/4C uncooked barley
Water
Slow cooker

Place whole chicken in slow cooker and two of the whole celery stalks with the bullion and can of stock. Cover to top of chicken with water. Cook on high all day until you are ready for bed, then put it in the refrigerator overnight.

-->

The following day skim off the chilled fat at the top of the pot and pour the rest into a large stock pot through a strainer. The strainer catches the meat, bones and celery, while the pot catches the stock.

Separate the meat from the bones, discarding the bones in a safe place, away from your household pets reach and remove the celery, discarding this as well.

Once you are sure every tiny bone is out of your soup as well as the skin (don't put that in the soup please; it's not pleasant), then shred the chicken with your hands and put it back into the slow cooker along with the broth.

Now you add your carrots, chopped celery and barley.

Place the pot back on high heat for 2-3 hours then turn the temperature down to low for the rest of the day. When you come home, you can eat this soup.

Put it back in the refrigerator overnight after dinner and cook it again on low the following day. This is going to turn your amazing soup into creamed soup!! Even better! The barley thickens the soup.

Put this into individual serving sized containers that you can readily heat. I put some in the refrigerator for the week and the rest in the freezer for another time.

TBLT

2 slices whole grain, low carb bread (17-18 total gms.) {Toasted if you like}
2 slices (TB) Turkey Bacon
Lots of lettuce (whatever kind you like)
1tsp. coconut oil to "butter" the bread
Sprinkle of Mrs. Dash, Original
1 small tomato
Build your sandwich, saving a couple of tomato slices for the side. This makes you eat slower and feel like you are eating more.

When you eat any meal, try to take a small bite, put the food down on the plate, enjoy the flavor as you chew, then take a sip of water and breathe. It's not a race. Repeat this process throughout your meal and it will last longer, making you feel more satisfied. You will actually fill up faster as well once you get used to this way of eating.

Bagel & Cream Cheese

Doesn't the sound of that make your mouth water? I love bagels and thought I couldn't eat them, but I have found a way to even enjoy this.
*Choose whole grain or whole wheat bagels.
½ bagel, toasted if you prefer (I like the crunch)
2T low fat cream cheese (my favorite is the vegetable)
Sprinkle of cinnamon (this is for its health benefits)

Can I tell you how incredibly satisfying 2 whole Tablespoons of this cream cheese is? It's decadent. Enjoy a nice slow cup of tea or coffee with this.

Nibble, sip, breathe; nibble, sip, breathe. I try to spend at least 15 minutes on each meal. Enjoy your time eating, whether with others or alone.

Veggie Bake

You can use any vegetables you like, but be sure to check carb counts. Zucchini and yellow squash are quite low, so I can indulge in a large portion of this. The combinations are endless.

Zucchini

Yellow squash

Peppers, red and green

Grape tomatoes

Coconut oil

Shredded parmesan cheese

*Cut up all the veggies and use the amounts you like. If you like zucchini best, use more of that. Drizzle melted coconut oil lightly over the vegetable and toss with Mrs. Dash, original. Bake at 350°F for 20 minutes in a deep pan. Stir and sprinkle with cheese before baking in the oven for about a half hour or until tender. Do not overcook or it will be mushy and unappetizing. I eat one cup of this for a serving. Notice I went easy on the tomatoes because of their higher carb count.

French Toast & Pears

1 Jumbo egg + 1/4C egg whites

2 slices low carb, whole grain bread (17-18gm carbs)

½ pear

1t cinnamon

1/2T raw bran

1T vanilla soy milk

1/4C Sugar Free maple syrup

1/2t butter (optional)

2 slices turkey bacon

Mix eggs, cinnamon, bran and milk together. Dip bread, both sides in this mixture and cook in a skillet for a couple of minutes per side, until egg is cooked through. Dot with butter.

Saute pears in pan with 1T water until tender, then add syrup to pan to heat. Serve with turkey bacon and savor every bite.

Enjoying Fruit

I incorporate one piece of fruit into every day. I may have ½ a
piece of fruit with my breakfast, like the French toast and ½ a
piece of fruit with some cheese later in the day. There are
vitamins and fiber in the fruits that your body needs, but keep in
mind the carb counts, as always. More is not better in the case of a
diabetic program.

After cutting my fruit in ½ I store the other ½ ready to go in a
baggie in the fridge. Try not to cut too much fruit ahead as it
browns. That being said, there are convenient packs at the store
now of pre-portioned, sliced fruits. I usually pick up a package of
apples.
Some stores have pre-sliced strawberries, cantaloupe, honeydew
melon and other fruits that are great time savers. Use some
strawberries with your French toast one day. The strawberries
have a pretty low carb count, (3gms. for 1/4 cup) so enjoy.

Roast Beast Sandwich

4 oz. lean, low sodium, roast beef
Lots of lettuce
1-2 t ketchup
1 oz. cheese (I like low fat American)
2 slices whole grain or whole wheat (17-18gm carb) bread
   *If you want rye bread or toast, use one slice cut in ½

Cucumbers & drizzle of dressing on the side

Tuna Salad

A great way to amp up the vitamins is to add spinach to this salad. Here's what I did.

1C chopped iceberg lettuce (you can use any lettuce you like)
1/2C raw baby spinach
¼ small tomato, sliced
¼-1/2 C chopped cucumbers, with skin on and seeds removed
    (you can eat the seeds if you want to)
1 6oz can solid white tuna in water, drained (this makes it 5 oz. of tuna)
1 measured T of olive oil mayonnaise
Sprinkle of Mrs. Dash, original
*Mix the tuna, mayo and seasoning together/put over the salad.
On the side, I added ½ of a peach, sliced. Use whatever fruit you like. Blueberries are really nice with this dish and, if eaten one at a time, really make you feel like you are eating so much more.

Wrap It Up

Here's another way to enjoy some roast beef. When I shop, I buy one pound of a meat that week at the deli, always searching for the sales and low sodium or store roasted products. This is an opportunity to use these meats in many different ways, rather than buying many different meats each week and wasting them at the end of the week. Use what's left in your quiche at the end of the week.

Here I've used 4oz. roast beef, 2 tsp. ketchup, lettuce, 1 oz. cheese and 1 low carb tomato basil whole wheat wrap. Make your sandwich and slice on the diagonal.

Add ½ a piece of fruit or some tomatoes on the side. I have ½ a nectarine here.

As always, take your time and enjoy!

Banana Bread & Coffee

1T Cinnamon	1 ¼ C ripe mashed bananas
1 1/3 C Whole Wheat Flour	(about 4)
1 t Baking powder	1/3 C vanilla soy milk
½ t baking soda	1 T coconut oil, melted
Pinch of salt	2 t vanilla extract
¼ C Truvia	¼ C chopped walnuts or
3 T Raw Wheat Bran	almonds
1 T ground flax seed	¼ C Sugar free Chocolate Chips
	1 T raw, flaked coconut

Mix all ingredients together and pour into loaf pan, sprayed with coconut oil. Bake at 350∘F for 40 minutes or until a knife inserted into center comes out clean.

Serving size is 1/8 of the loaf.

I serve this with a nice hot cup of coffee or tea.

Apple Compote

This is one of the fruit compotes I like to use over French toast. You can use it in many other ways as well, including as a mix in for your oatmeal. If you mix it into the oatmeal, only use ¼ cup serving. On the French toast, ½ cup is sufficient. Here's what to do.

1 apple, chopped
1/2 C sugar free maple syrup
1 t cinnamon
1 t butter
2 T water

Cook the apple in a skillet for a few minutes, then add the water to steam, and swirl the apples in the pan, briefly. Add the cinnamon and cook until the apples still have a little bite left to them and the water has evaporated.

Add your butter and syrup to the pan and cook just until the butter melts. Yummy!

Fruit & Cheese

Who doesn't love a fruit and cheese platter? For us, however, it is not an appetizer, but a meal. I would not have this and then a meal and a dessert. We need to spread out our meals according to our individual time lines.

For this meal, use 1 oz. of your favorite cheese, cubed. Change up the cheese from time to time so you don't get bored and you can explore the amazing flavors offered.
Also add 1 serving of fruit. Here I decided on1 Cup of sugar melon. That's about 14 grams of carbs.

Try to choose the fruits that are in season whenever possible. I go to the farm when they are open. Don't be afraid to sniff the fruit (and tomatoes). If they smell sweet or like the fruit or veg. they should smell like, they are the ones you want. They will have the best flavor. It's your kitchen; make choices you will love.

Weird Combinations

Of course it's best to plan your meals, having carb, lean protein, healthy fat and veg.; but that's not always possible. Although this was not the best choice, it worked in a pinch. I had 1 small ear of corn, ½ a medium tomato and 2 slices of bacon.

The bacon was left over from breakfast one day and the corn from a dinner. I just had to heat and serve. Since there was already fat in the bacon, I sprayed my corn with butter flavored spray. This meal was satisfying and delicious, but keep in mind, these types of meals are not meant to be eaten often. Turkey bacon would've been better and perhaps a salad added.

Learning how to recognize what is in food is key. When you look at a meal, for instance, what do you see? In the past my answer would've been meat and vegetables for something like the bacon, corn and tomatoes. Now, my trained eye sees carbs, protein and fat.

See the difference? Even further than that I see high carb and high fat, which is why this would not be a choice I would often have.

The bacon is high fat, there are carbs in the tomatoes, which is why I don't count them as a veg and the same for the corn. Corn on the cob is very high in carbs, so go easy on it and please don't slather it in high fat butter and douse it in salt, which raises your blood pressure and in turn, your glucose levels. Salt is best left at the store. There's already a lot of salt in that bacon.

Take some time looking at food magazines or cookbooks and see if you can identify the carbs, fats, vegetable and proteins in the pictures. This is not a waste of time. It will help you plan your plates and recognize foods at a party.

The perfect plate is ½ filled with no carb vegetables, ¼ filled with carbs and ¼ filled with lean protein, with a small amount of good, healthy fat. The fat may be in a piece of fish or meat or on your vegetable or carbs or even on your salad. Look for hidden fat and salt.

Roasted Red Beet Chips

You cook these the same way you cooked the yellow beet chip recipe.

I wear gloves when making this dish because the red beets are very messy to work with.

Carrots can also be made into chips!

Experience with different root vegetables and have fun with it. As always, count those carbs.

SPAGHETTI SQUASH HEAVEN

If you haven't tried this, now's your chance. Cut a spaghetti squash in half, lengthwise and scoop out the pulp and seeds. Discard the pulp and cook the seeds the same as any squash. Spray the cut side with extra virgin olive oil and bake cut side down in a 350°F oven for about 20-25 minutes or until a knife goes in and comes out easily. Don't overcook and end up with mush. The skin will be slightly browned. Gently scrape out insides with a fork and fluff.

From here, your options are endless. I chose to add meatballs and marinara sauce with crumbled spicy sausage. Go easy on the sauce and shaved parmesan cheese. 1 serving would be about 1 Cup of squash with ¼ cup sauce and 1 ½ meatballs cut in half and ¼ cup crumbled sausage. 1 T of shaved parm. on top.

Alternative:
1 Cup squash
¼ cup peas or snap peas
¼ cup ricotta cheese
½ cup cooked ground turkey

Turkey Sandwich

Can I just tell you how much I love my sandwiches! I'm so glad I found a bread that I can eat 2 slices of and really enjoy. They're out there. Start reading labels.

This sandwich is simply 4 oz. store roasted turkey breast, 1 oz. sharp American cheese,
A hunk of lettuce leaves, 1 teaspoon of coconut oil on the bread, a sprinkle of Mrs. Dash original and 2 slices of low carb multi-grain bread, toasted.
I've added ½ an apple, sliced on the side. Who needs chips? I honestly do not miss them!

Find the foods that fit into your meal plan that have the highest amount of flavor and you will not miss the junk food as much. Instead of thinking what you can't eat, focus on what you are eating and enjoy every bite of it.

TURKEY & STUFFING

My favorite meal is turkey dinner, but I especially like the stuffing. Here I have made a diabetic friendly version of stuffing I'd like to share with you,

1 Box Stove Top Whole Wheat Stuffing Mix
7-8 slices whole grain or whole wheat bread, cut into chunks
3 slices store roasted deli turkey, chopped
5 large button mushrooms, chopped
1 crushed bouillon cube

--→

½ C homemade gravy if you have it, or 1/2C chicken stock (low sodium)
1T butter, melted
1/2T dried rosemary
1/4C dried cranberries
2-3C warm water (enough to moisten all the bread and have the stuffing come together. If you need more water, use more.)
1/2C cooked onions

Mix all ingredients together and stuff into turkey. When you baste your turkey, baste the stuffing that sticks out as well. The stuffing inside is getting drippings through the top of the turkey, which will flavor it further. When the turkey comes out of the oven, I put the stuffing in another pan and cook it until crisp on top.

Your serving size will be about a ½ a cup. It's sooooo delicious!

For the turkey, cook it for the length of time recommended on the label, but be sure to baste it with the pan drippings every hour. This makes the moistest turkey ever! The downside of basting is that it adds fat to your turkey, but it's worth it....just have a smaller portion.

Since you already have a carb with the stuffing have some green beans and just a hint of the gravy if you want. Leave the rest to the guests.

SUGAR FREE BOSTON CRÈME PIE

Prepare and bake one box Sugar Free Vanilla cake mix according to package.

Cool cake completely, then cut in half, lengthwise.

Fill with 4 ready-made sugar free vanilla pudding cups; put the top of the cake back on. Put cake back in fridge to cool while you do the next step.

In microwave safe bowl mix 1 bag sugar free chocolate chips + 3/4C light cream.

Microwave for 2 minutes then stir until blended and creamy. Put in fridge to cool for about 15 minutes. (Too long and it won't flow; too short and it will melt your cream filling and spill all over the cake.)

Gently spread chocolate in light layer over the top of the cake only. Put cake and extra chocolate back in the fridge to cool for about 20 minutes.

Take the cake back out and gently add the rest of the chocolate to the top/middle of the cake. It will spill down naturally, but if it doesn't , coax it gently to the sides. Decorate as you like.
**This is sugar free, but not calorie or carb free. Please only have about a 12th of the cake for a serving and only after 2-3 hours after a meal; not right after. Enjoy this, but only on occasion. This is not a good choice for a daily meal. Make it special, just like you.

Small Meal Ideas:

1. 1/4C unsalted nuts + ½ pear

2. 1 oz. cheese + 3 dried apricots + ½ C snap peas

3. ½ banana + 1 T Peanut butter

4. 1 sugar free pudding cup + ½ banana + 1 T sugar free whipped cream

5. 1 glucose balancing granola bar

6. 4 stalks celery + 2 T chunky peanut butter (low sugar)

7. ½ C berries + 1 T sugar free whipped cream

8. 1 clementine + 1 oz. cheese

9. 1 C cucumber slices + 1 T low fat, low salt dressing

10. 1 hardboiled egg + 4 wholegrain, low fat, low sodium crackers

*Now it's your turn. Add to this list and keep it handy. I've given you the tools to begin, now it's up to you. Work with your medical team and figure the rest out for yourself using these rules and remembering to test and count.

You CAN do this!

I was diagnosed on February 28, 2015 and at the close of this book, it is now October 26th, 2015. Eight months have passed and I have gone from a level 9 A1C to a 5.8 A1C. I am one point away from my goal, according to my doctor of 5.7, which takes me out of the pre-diabetic realm and into the norm.

I've also lost 45 pounds to date. My blood pressure is perfect, my good and bad cholesterol levels are perfect and I'm feeling so much better.

Just because my numbers are really good, does not mean I can stop. My body has the potential to go back to diabetic levels at any time. I need to keep eating and exercising and adjusting all this as needed in order to stay healthy and live longer. I'm always learning. I'm with you and so is God.

I cannot stress enough that I am not a doctor or a nutritionist. I am not telling you what to do with your body, only telling you what I have done, that worked for me.
This is your walk and you and your medical team alone can determine what the best path for you is.

I hope that what I've learned and am passing on to you helps and proves to be a good tool for you to add to your toolbox.

I pray that all who pick up this book, are blessed with a healthier, more active and joyful life.

Never give up. Take it one step at a time and don't be overwhelmed. It gets easier. Trust me.

Blessings, Love and Peace to you and your family.

Roberta

www.ingramcontent.com/pod-product-compliance
Lightning Source LLC
Chambersburg PA
CBHW081725270326
41933CB00017B/3297